FEAR OF PREMENSTRUAL SYNDROME (PMS)

&

Managing your first period: Tips for girls with ADHD

Dr. Pamela Hutson.

1

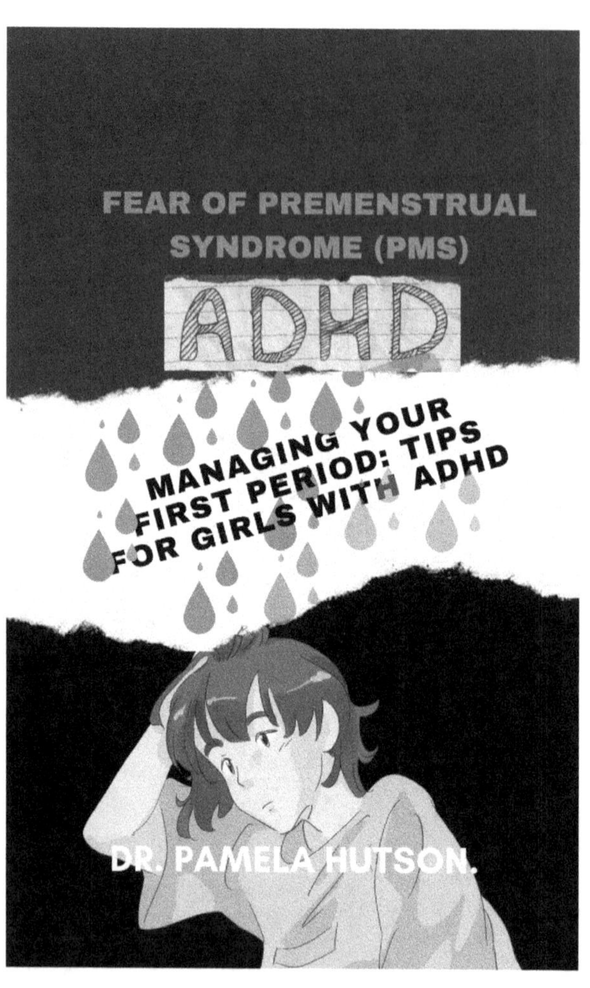

FEAR OF PREMENSTRUAL SYNDROME (PMS)
ADHD
MANAGING YOUR FIRST PERIOD: TIPS FOR GIRLS WITH ADHD
DR. PAMELA HUTSON.

Table of content

Having been a mother of 2 girls and working in the hospital for over a decade now, PMS is one of the major issues suffered by most American women and girls.

I was a victim to it too, having attended to so many people who had PMS this book was written basically for managing PMS.

People with ADHD are more likely to suffer from PMS.

INTRODUCTION

PMS symptoms include mood swings, irritability, lateness in the breasts, increased hunger, nausea, back pain, and fainting. It is clear from some of these symptoms that **PMS** generally has a negative influence on teenagers' productivity. This includes a poor performance at work, suicidal sentiments, and even the impulse to harm oneself or others might be brought on by depression. Consequently, there is a condition when a person experiences morning anger, anxiety, and/or sadness. Depression, rage, and other negative emotions often occur, and they may have an impact on an individual or their surroundings.

The prevalence of **PMS** is between 70 and 90 percent in America, 61 to 85 percent in Sweden, 51.2% in Morocco, 85 in Australia, 95 in Japan, and 73 percent in Taiwan.

According to studies, at least 50% of women suffer **PMS**, according to Knight's 2004 report. In the same way, up to 90% of American women of reproductive age have been said to have PMS symptoms. The results of a poll of 242 students at Jimma University in Ethiopia, who had an average age of 20, revealed that 99.6% of respondents had PMS. Premenstrual dysphoric disorder was observed to affect 27% of the participants; 14% often skipped class; 15% were unable to take tests due to their PMS.

Overall research reveals that **PMS** is a prevalent kind of disease encountered by teens throughout Asia. In Iran, it was shown that about 98.2% of students had mild or moderate **PMS**. In Sri Lanka, 65.7% of young women suffer from PMS (American College of Obstetricians and Gynecologists). The incidence rate in Indonesia is between 70 and 90 percent (Ernawati, 2012).

Women's nutritional state is a factor that contributes to PMS.

Other reasons include those brought on by serotonin malfunction, psychological issues, societal issues, and hormonal imbalance. Menarche (first menstruation) in teenage females is significantly influenced by their dietary status.

Adolescents who have **PMS** may work less efficiently while doing everyday tasks. Teenagers' performance at school may be impacted by PMS symptoms. In a 2011 research with hsCRP levels of 1.70% of women, as many as seven respondents reported having mild PMS. Conversely, among those with hs-CRP levels >1, 70% of respondents with severe PMS had a waist circumference of 8 and a body mass index of 8. PMS is at risk when the hs-CRP level is five times higher (IK: 2,155-204,614). There is a risk of STDs even if the waist circumference is five times higher (CI: 1,039-28,533). Based on prior research, this study focuses on respondents who had severe PMS and a normal BMI of 30%. On the other hand, severe PMS affected 70% of the 15 responders with obese BMIs.

Thirty percent of the six individuals with normal waist circumferences who obtained waist circumference measurements experienced severe PMS. Find out how the hormone estrogen affects teenage girls who have premenstrual syndrome among the 14 obese respondents.

<u>WHAT IS PREMENSTRUAL SYNDROME (PMS)?</u>

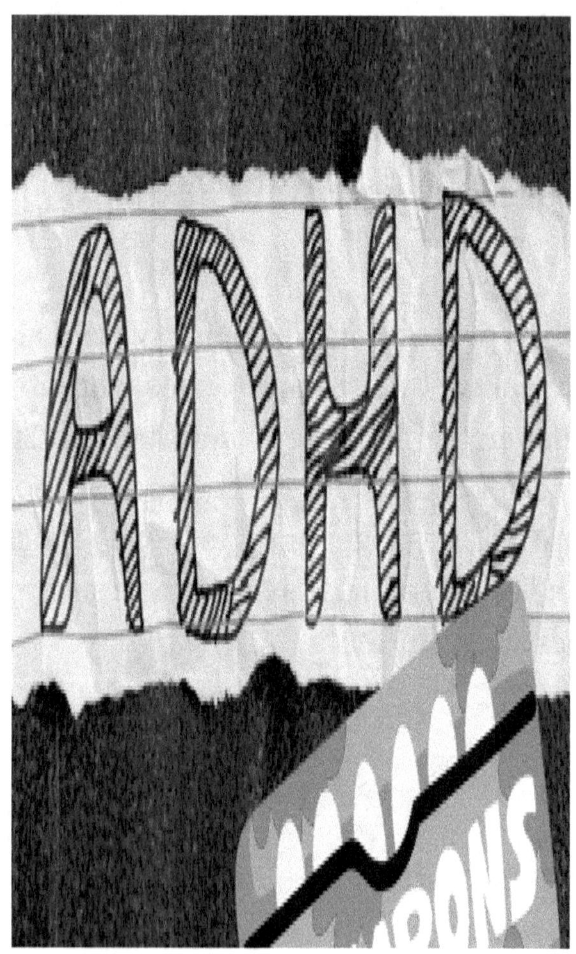

You can experience bloating, headaches, mood swings, or other physical and emotional changes a week or two before the onset of your period. Premenstrual syndrome, or **PMS**, is the term for these cyclical symptoms. **PMS** affects women to varying degrees in about 85% of cases. Some people experience more severe symptoms known as premenstrual dysphoric disorder, which can interfere with work or personal relationships.

A girl experiencing hormonal imbalance, edema, or cramps can't or won't notice it. It can be difficult for girls who also have **ADHD**.
Periods are distracting for everyone, but for females with attention-deficit hyperactivity

disorder, managing periods and **ADHD** can be particularly challenging. Girls with **ADHD** frequently lack the attentional bandwidth necessary to deal with things like cramping, mood swings, and remembering to pack tampons or change their pads regularly.

No matter how long you've had your period, whether it's been a year or ten, it never stops being disruptive. A female experiencing hormonal imbalance, puffiness, or cramps can't help but notice it. It can be particularly challenging for girls who already have **ADHD**.
ADHD and **PMS** don't get along very well. This is especially true the week before the start of menstruation. Dopamine declines as progesterone rise. As a result, these girls may become more agitated, forgetful, and emotional, intensifying their **ADHD** symptoms.

Why Does PMS Occur?

Although the precise cause of **PMS** is unknown, we do know that the week before your period, estrogen and progesterone levels decrease. Many medical professionals think that this drop in hormone levels is what sets off **PMS** symptoms. Alterations in the brain's chemical composition or a lack of specific vitamins and minerals could also be at fault. The symptoms could also worsen if you consume too much salt, alcohol, or caffeine.

Who Suffers from PMS?

Any woman who gets a period may have **PMS**, however, some are more susceptible to the condition:

- In the late 20s to mid-40s, PMS is more prevalent.
- PMS is often more intense in older teenagers compared to younger teens.
- In your 40s, PMS could be more severe.

- PMS is more common in women who have had at least one pregnancy.
- PMS symptoms may worsen in women with a history of depression or another mood condition.

Symptoms of PMS

Premenstrual syndrome symptoms might be more difficult to deal with than the actual period for **PMS** Girls with **ADHD**, who frequently find it difficult to control their emotions even under the finest circumstances. The ups and downs of PMS can sometimes be more severe for girls with **ADHD,** according to clinical psychologist Mandi Silverman, PsyD. It can be really overwhelming for a girl who already struggles to control her emotions because it is so distracting. Unfortunately, PMS is a common occurrence for many girls. But it doesn't imply it has to be a recurring nightmare.

Everyone experiences premenstrual syndrome differently. Some females may experience the same symptoms every month regardless of their hormonal state, while others may experience the same symptoms every month regardless of their hormonal state.
Some of the popular symptoms may include

❖ **Cravings**
Cravings When **PMS** comes, many women have unique cravings, often for salty or sweet foods like chocolate cake. The causes of this are not entirely apparent. Some women can experience nausea or a loss of appetite. Constipation and bloating are also typical.

❖ Acne

One of the most prevalent symptoms of **PMS** is acne, which doesn't only affect teens. Skin glands may create more sebum in response to hormonal changes. This greasy material may clog the pores and cause a breakout, which will be apparent and serve as a visual cue that your period is approaching.

❖ Pain

Several different types of aches and pains, including

- backache

- Headaches
- supple breasts
- aching joints

❖ Mood swings

The worst aspect of PMS for many women is its unexpected effect on mood. On and off, you may experience irritability, rage, weeping fits, melancholy, and anxiety in the days before your period. Some women may have memory loss and attention problems during this period.

The greatest way to help your daughter deal with the unpleasant sensations brought on by **PMS**, according to Dr. Silverman, is to assist her in being ready. A few months of tracking her symptoms can help rule out external causes. Some of the symptoms can be lessened for some girls by increasing their sleep, changing their diet, or moving more. Have her make a chart showing the effects of her period over three cycles, advises Dr. Silverman. "Once your daughter starts to recognize how her cycle affects her, she'll be able to make beneficial changes so she can be better prepared for things like lack of focus or moodiness that consistently cause problems," the expert said. You may decide she'll record the lectures that week and watch them again when she's feeling more focused, for instance, if her period makes it even harder to focus in class.

Add more physical activities to her routine if she feels better in the months when she exercises more. If she feels happier when she sleeps more, suggest giving an earlier bedtime a try for a week.

She will experience less stress and a greater chance of completing assignments on time if she begins work on papers or projects that are due during or shortly after her period.

Encourage her to skip making arrangements with friends during those few days each month if PMS makes her feel worn out or too emotional. She can then get some rest and stay away from any awkward social settings until she feels better.

ESTROGEN AND HOW IT AFFECTS PMS

Estrogen is primarily to blame for persons with **ADHD** experiencing such difficulty during their cycle. Estrogen can activate particular populations of dopamine and serotonin receptors in the brain, according to Pharmacological Reviews. These compounds' concentrations in the brain decrease when estrogen levels do in the weeks preceding a period. Numerous of the same substances have an impact on **ADHD** symptoms.

As a result, people with **ADHD** may be more susceptible to estrogen, and their symptoms may and generally do worsen throughout the month as hormone levels change.

What is Estrogen?

An essential sex hormone for maintaining sexual and reproductive health is estrogen. Your natural cycle of menstruation and menopause causes changes in your estrogen levels. Estrogen levels that are consistently high or low can indicate a problem that needs to be addressed by your doctor.

Description of estrogen.

One of the two sex hormones that are frequently linked to cisgender women, transgender men, and nonbinary people with vaginal organs is estrogen. Estrogen, along with progesterone, is essential for the health of your reproductive system. Estrogen has a role in the development of secondary sex traits (such as breasts, hips, etc.), menstruation, pregnancy, and menopause.

Additionally, estrogen is crucial to other bodily systems. Because of this, while AFAB people produce the most estrogen, both genders do as well.

What variations of estrogen are there?

Estrogen comes in three main forms:

1. The main form of estrogen that your body produces after menopause is estrogen (E1).
2. During your reproductive years, the main type of estrogen in your body is estradiol (E2). It is the strongest estrogenic type.
3. During pregnancy, the main type of estrogen is estriol (E3).

FUNCTION

What part does estrogen play in a woman's or DFAB's reproductive health?
Like all hormones, estrogen is a chemical messenger. It instructs the body on when to initiate and end procedures that have an impact on your sexual and reproductive health. Your body goes through these procedures and changes significantly.

Puberty

During puberty, estrogen levels increase. Breast size and general body composition change as a result of the increase, which affects secondary sex traits (like curves).

Periodic period

Estrogen is a key player in your menstrual cycle, along with progesterone and hormones produced in your brain (FSH and LH). Your cycles will remain regular because of the precise balance between these hormones. When your ovaries release an egg, a process known as ovulation, estrogen plays a role. It also thickens the endometrium, the lining of your uterus, preparing it for pregnancy.

Childbirth & Fertility

In the days before ovulation, estrogen peaks. Your most fertile time is right now. The cervical mucus in your throat thins as a result of estrogen use, making it easier for sperm to pass through and reach an egg for fertilization. If you have sexual contact, these estrogen-induced alterations make it simpler for you to get pregnant.

The presence of estrogen makes having sex more comfortable regardless of where you are in your menstrual cycle. It lessens pain from penetrative intercourse by maintaining thick, elastic, and lubricated vaginal walls.

Menopause

During perimenopause, the period just before menopause, estrogen levels decline. Before menopause, the perimenopause may extend several years. When you go a full 12 months without getting your period, menopause officially starts. Around age 51 is when it typically occurs. Your estrogen levels fall throughout menopause, and you stop ovulating. Night sweats, hot flashes, mood swings, and vaginal dryness are just a few symptoms that could result from a drop in estrogen levels.

During menopause, your body switches from producing estradiol (E2) to estrone (E1) as the main estrogen.

What part does estrogen play in men's or AMAB's reproductive health?

Male at birth (AMAB) individuals' reproductive health is also impacted by estrogen. Estrogen affects sex drive, erection ability, and sperm production in nonbinary people with penises, transgender women, and cisgender men.

Low sex drive might result from low estrogen levels. Erectile dysfunction and infertility might result from having too much of it. Breast enlargement, or gynecomastia, can be brought on by too much estrogen.

If you were given the gender of a man at birth and are worried about your estrogen levels, you should seek advice from an endocrinologist or a functional medicine specialist.

What is estrogen's non-reproductive purpose?
Your skeletal, cardiovascular, and central neurological systems are regulated by

estrogen in ways that have an impact on your general health. How estrogen impacts:

- degrees of cholesterol.
- levels of blood sugar.
- muscle and bone mass.
- blood flow and circulation.
- Skin hydration and collagen production.
- brain activity, including your capacity for concentration.

ANATOMY

Where in the body does estrogen reside? During your reproductive years, your ovaries produce the majority of your estrogen. Adipose tissue (body fat) and your adrenal glands, which are located in your kidneys, both secrete estrogen. During pregnancy, the placenta, which is the organ that permits the sharing of nutrients between the mother and the fetus, secretes estrogen.

Once estrogen is released, it moves via your bloodstream to the area of your body that needs to be activated. There, estrogen interacts with an estrogen receptor protein to initiate the process. Your entire body contains estrogen receptors.

DISEASES AND CONDITIONS

Which frequent diseases and disorders are linked to estrogen?

The majority of illnesses that fall under the category of women's health include estrogen. Among the most typical are:

Anorexia nervosa: Low estrogen levels are linked to disorders like anorexia nervosa. Period irregularities and missed periods might result from low estrogen levels (amenorrhea). Little estrogen may also be seen in those who have very low body fat (such as models or athletes) or who have eating disorders.

Increased estrogen exposure does not raise the chance of developing breast cancer, according to studies, but it may make the disease worse after it has already started.

Endometriosis: Although estrogen doesn't cause endometriosis, it can make the discomfort associated with it worse. Falling estrogen levels can result in physical and emotional changes that reduce the pleasure of sex, which is referred to as female sexual dysfunction (FSD). The use of estrogen for hormone replacement is not recommended until menopause.

Fibrocystic breasts: Your breast tissue may feel lumpy, sensitive, or unpleasant due to fluctuating estrogen levels throughout your menstrual cycle.

Low and high estrogen levels might mess with your menstrual cycle, resulting in infertility. Infertility may be correlated with underlying factors that might result in low and high estrogen levels.

Obesity: Women with higher levels of body fat frequently have higher levels of estrogen.

Osteoporosis: When your bones are weak, they are more likely to fracture and break. PCOS is a condition that develops when the ovaries create an excessive amount of androgens (hormones associated with being assigned male at birth). Estrogen levels can occasionally be excessively high in PCOS when compared to progesterone levels. Premature menopause is another name for the syndrome known as primary ovarian insufficiency, which causes the ovaries to abruptly stop releasing eggs (before age 40). Your ovaries therefore fail to secrete the amount of estrogen that your body requires. The cyclical hormone changes related to menstruation can cause uncomfortable physical symptoms and emotional changes, which are known as premenstrual syndrome (PMS) and premenstrual dysphoric disorder (PMDD). PMS and PMDD may be brought on by drops in estrogen after ovulation.

Ovaries are frequently undeveloped in Turner syndrome, which lowers estrogen levels. As a result, those who have this illness might not have their periods or develop breasts.

Endometrial cancer, often known as uterine cancer, can develop when the lining of the uterus thickens due to high estrogen levels. Cancer cells may eventually begin to multiply.

Fibroids and polyps in the uterus: Excess estrogen may be linked to non-cancerous tumors known as fibroids or polyps that develop in the uterus.

Atrophic vaginitis, also known as vaginal atrophy, is a condition where the lining of your vagina thins and becomes dry due to a lack of estrogen. Most women experience vaginal shrinkage throughout menopause and postmenopause.

The influence of estrogen on ailments that affect other bodily systems is still being studied. For instance, gastrointestinal illnesses and several endocrine abnormalities have both been associated with estrogen.

What is the average level of estrogen?
Estrogen levels fluctuate during the course of a lifetime. The variation is typical. For instance, it is typical for estrogen levels to increase during adolescence and decrease as menopause approaches. Estrogen levels often increase during ovulation so that your body can get ready for pregnancy. When the pregnancy alterations are unnecessary, it's typical for levels to drop throughout your period.

Consistently low or high levels could be an indication of an underlying problem that needs your doctor's attention.

What occurs when estrogen levels remain low over time?

Low estrogen levels are frequently a warning sign that menopause is just around the corner. Low estrogen may also be a symptom of Turner syndrome, infertility issues, nutritional deficiencies, etc.

Some signs could be:
- breast sensitivity
- brittle or weak bones.
- sweating at night and hot flashes.
- No periods or irregular periods.
- headaches and difficulty focusing.
- fatigue, sleepiness, and sleep disturbances.
- sadness, impatience, and mood swings.
- Dryness of the vagina causes unpleasant sexual encounters (dyspareunia).

What results from persistently high estrogen levels?

Numerous problems, including polyps, fibroids, PCOS, endometriosis discomfort, ovarian tumors, etc., might be linked to an excess of estrogen in the body. Your levels could be elevated as a result of having too much estrogen in comparison to progesterone, the second sex hormone. You can end up with too much estrogen in your body as a result of the medications you're taking that contain it.

Some signs could be:
- reduced sex motivation
- gaining weight, especially around the waist and hips.
- irregular cycles (unpredictable timing, light or heavy bleeding).
- PMS or PMDD symptoms that are getting worse.
- How can I determine my estrogen level?

- Your levels of estrone (E1), estradiol (E2), or estriol can be determined by an estrogen test (E3). Your doctor will take a quick blood sample, which will then be sent to a lab for evaluation.

What prevalent disorders related to estrogen are treated?

Low estrogen is frequently treated with hormone replacement therapy (HT), especially in menopausal women. Your doctor may recommend a combination of estrogen and progesterone or tiny doses of estrogen to increase your level when you have HT (or the synthetic version of progesterone, progestin). However, HT has hazards and isn't suitable for everyone. Whether you are a good candidate for HT should be discussed with your physician.

CARE

How can I keep my estrogen levels in check?

Sometimes it's impossible to avoid the ailments brought on by hormonal imbalances. Nevertheless, you can adopt healthy habits to support preserving your general well-being.

Get adequate rest. Each night, getting enough restful sleep is beneficial for your body's ability to maintain the balanced hormone levels required for carrying out vital processes.
Maintain stress control. Your body may overproduce the stress chemicals cortisol and adrenaline in response to high levels of stress. Your estrogen levels may be adversely affected by an overabundance of stress hormones.

The appropriate quantity of exercise You can control how much you eat and how much body fat you have by getting a reasonable quantity of activity. You may sleep better as a result of it.

Reduce your alcohol consumption. Your estrogen levels may increase if you drink. Too much estrogen exposure over time may increase your risk of developing cancer. Develop healthy eating habits. To help your hormones balance, keep an eye on your dietary intake. Hormone balance can be improved by cutting back on sugary meals and increasing fiber and healthy fats (such as those found in fish, olive oil, nuts, and seeds).
Cleveland Clinic's statement

Your reproductive system's health, as well as your general health, depends on estrogen. Your estrogen levels will naturally change with age and menstrual cycle. You may suffer unpleasant symptoms that are worth discussing with your doctor if they are consistently high or low. There are treatments that can help, most frequently in the form of hormone medications following menopause, lifestyle changes, or contraception.

THE ADHD MIND IN ACTION

How the Menstrual Cycle Intensifies PMS and ADHD

ADHD and PMS have a tumultuous connection. A person's productivity and focus may increase in lockstep with her estrogen during the second week of her cycle as a result of hormonal changes during the menstrual cycle. Then, as estrogen levels fall and PMS sets in after ovulation, the humming machine grinds to a halt. Progesterone levels rise and dopamine levels fall during the week before menstruation, which can exacerbate emotional dysregulation and trigger ADHD symptoms like impulsivity, forgetfulness, and impatience.

Recently, it has been discovered that during a typical 30-day cycle, the menstrual cycle has both positive and negative effects on ADHD symptoms. Do you have periods of

the month when your symptoms of ADHD
go better or worse?

For some people, the three days prior to
period are the most detrimental to working
memory. They might enter the kitchen 100
times because they can't recall what they are
doing. I've always been afraid that after
estrogen levels decline between
perimenopause and menopause, people
won't be able to hide their symptoms at
work, which will make it harder for me to
have a career.

Others observe a variation in their capacity
to control their attention as they progress
through a cycle. When they are in the
middle of a cycle, they find it simpler to be
mindful. The closer I go to period, the more
likely they are to forget things or lose focus.

Some people's ADHD symptoms worsen in
the week before their period.

Energy levels drop, distractibility rises, and executive functioning deteriorates. The majority of people tend to be totally inattentive at work. When they see where they are in their cycle on the calendar, it will finally click for them.

Different opinions were gathered from several people who shared how managing ADHD has been for them. For safety reasons, the names of these people were not published. Read from them how they it feels like to them and how they usually manage to survive;

"I notice that as my first week's (flow) symptoms lessen, my ADHD symptoms are so much better - I do so much more on those days," she said. I'm more intellectually capable, stable, and motivated. However, my symptoms get worse the closer ovulation gets. I'm more agitated and have trouble concentrating. The symptoms then dreadfully subside just before my flow, when I can hardly focus. I suffer a lot with motivation and emotional dysregulation, and I am even more forgetful. I feel bad for my spouse and children, who have to put up with my erratic behavior. I can now better comprehend what I go through after learning about the hormonal changes that occur during a woman's cycle. To minimize my symptoms, I'm still attempting to understand how to work with my body. I hope more research will be done to support people like myself who rely on hormone cycles to thrive rather than merely get by!

"The week before my period, I become more worried and have difficulties sleeping. Additionally, it's harder for me to focus, organize my thoughts, and maintain a schedule. Additionally, I am more emotional at work. I feel uncontrollable. I've learned how to manage my symptoms over the years, but once a month, I still have a bad case of the feels.

"My menstrual cycle and ADHD have both been challenging. I exaggerate everything I want to accomplish and can achieve during peak ovulation because I feel like a superhero. Then, when my period draws near, it starts to fade. I am a complete mess with no focus because of my emotional dysregulation. I make irrational decisions like quitting my job only to reflect a week later that it wasn't all that horrible.

"I have trouble controlling my emotions and impulses the day or two before my period. I find myself in circumstances when I binge eat and find it difficult to control my opinions, which causes conflict at home. As an OB-GYN nurse, I can attest to the fact that dopamine levels fall when progesterone levels are high. Therefore, the week before menstruation is a terrible time for women with ADHD to try and do anything.

"I endure mood dysregulation and throbbing headaches right before my period. I also have low arousal and a serious lack of motivation for a few days after my period.

"My ADHD would get so bad the week before my period that I couldn't do certain tasks for work, like correcting tests and figuring out students' grades. I'm relieved to be post-menopausal.

"A week before my period is scheduled to arrive, my mind turns to complete peanut butter. Focusing and staying on task are near impossible tasks. Peak sensory overload has occurred. The days are ruled by impatience, and I feel so overwhelmed.

"A week before the onset of my menstruation, my ADHD symptoms became worse. I'm more tense and disorganized. Nothing comes to mind! My worry can become out of control. I believe that I have more mental clarity when my period is over. I can complete tasks more quickly and easily, and I'm more "with it."

Oh my goodness, YES! PMS exacerbates typical ADHD symptoms including being easily distracted and too sensitive to touch and noise. Dishes being left out, the animals meowing, and my boyfriend touching me all aggravate me greatly.

"I have trouble speaking clearly right before and at the start of my period, or I can't come up with the correct words. I am a lot more emotional and forgetful. When I once forgot why I had entered the kitchen, I started crying. Before I read about it, I didn't really pay attention to how radically my mind

changes during my menstrual cycle, but now
I can't help but notice it.

GETTING READY FOR PMS WITH ADHD

A girl with ADHD may not be ready even though her period is regular and arrives on the same day and at the same time each month (pardon the pun). Unfortunately, one of the main problems for people with ADHD is forgetfulness. Additionally, it seems that the task's importance makes forgetting it simpler. Being ready will be very beneficial. It will be simpler for daughters when the time comes if mothers can assist them by planning ahead and doing so with and for them.

Among the strategies to get ready are:

- Put a phone reminder in place. If the daughter has a phone, she could do it on that as well. [Perhaps both]

- Ensure that there are enough supplies on hand.
- Putting school supplies in a little makeup bag
- Stock up on supplies for the night.

The First Period of Your Daughter: How To Handle It

The beginning of your daughter's period is a significant turning point. It's an important turning point when your daughter gets her first period. As a girl, it's important for her, and as a mother, it's a big day for you. When girls start having periods, it signals that puberty has fully begun and there is no turning back.

Even the most knowledgeable mothers may feel a little embarrassed and unable to handle this situation with grace during a period, but since you know it's coming, you can perfectly prepare for it.

Some females begin their period as early as 8 or 9 years old, while others may wait until they are 16 years old. Whatever age your daughter is when she begins to period, it is the appropriate time for her.

Periods have some genetic ties, so this shouldn't come as a complete surprise. Therefore, it is possible that your daughter will experience her first period at a similar age to when you did.

A year or two after the development of her breast buds is another indicator that your daughter might start her period soon. Your daughter is beginning to approach puberty, and her period may not be long after.

❖ **Start Discussing It Prior to It Occurring**

Given that you are the mother in this situation, there are various methods you might use to ease your daughter's first period. Consider the things that might have helped you during your first menstruation. Make sure your daughter is informed of the upcoming changes before they take place.

One of your responsibilities as a mother to a biological female is preparing her for these changes because getting your period as a young girl and not expecting it may be really distressing.
Talk to your daughter about what will happen to her body years before she is expected to get her period. Even if your daughter is just 5 years old when you start talking to her about periods, keep the conversation on a level that they will understand.
It's likely that your daughter will witness you using pads, or tampons, or experiencing cramps if you receive your period.

A menstruation can be simply explained in biological terms as the shedding of her uterine lining once a month. Tell them she has two ovaries and a uterus. One of her ovaries releases a little egg into our fallopian tubes during ovulation each month. An unfertilized egg will shed itself and some uterine lining before leaving the body through the vagina as blood.

A period is anticipated to last 3–7 days, and it typically starts off heavy before tapering off. Sticking to the facts regarding periods and the reasons we have them, advises WebMD.
Your daughter is approaching the reproductive years, so it's critical that she understands her monthly cycle and the likelihood of being pregnant.

Your daughter will know more the more you teach her. A period does not guarantee that your daughter will engage in sexual activity. She's probably years away from it, but too many women grow up not completely understanding their bodies.

❖ Build a Period Kit.

Create a tiny period pack for your daughter before her first period even arrives to make the transition to a new period even smoother. To capture the blood from their periods and prevent it from staining her clothes, your girl will need sanitary pads, napkins, or tampons.
Pads may be more convenient for younger girls until they are ready to use a tampon. Teach your daughter about the various sizes and levels of absorbency available in pads and tampons.

For sanitary purposes and to prevent pads and tampons from growing too full, they must be replaced every 3 to 4 hours.

Particularly when used for an extended period of time, tampons pose substantial dangers to girls and women and can result in toxic shock syndrome.

In case your girl gets cramps before or during her period, a pack can also contain a tiny warming pad or some ibuprofen. This kit can be concealed from her peers by being packed inside a compact makeup bag.

❖ **Be straightforward**

Please be careful not to attribute your unpleasant thoughts about periods to your daughter when she starts her period. She can feel terrified if she understands there will likely be a lot of blood and pain.
It makes no sense to make her dislike her period before it ever occurs because you won't know how periods affect her body until it really happens to her.

Ensure your daughter that she is able to perform all of her typical activities while having her period. Be involved and assist your daughter keep track of her menstrual cycle. The first few menstrual cycles may not be regular, which can only make matters worse.

Parenting has obviously advanced to a new stage, but it is manageable.
Your daughter may have learned that an average cycle lasts 28 days in health class.

However, she should anticipate that her first three periods would be somewhat erratic before settling into a hazy pattern.

She might have one and then go 2-3 months without having another, according to Holmes. When she has had three periods, they should begin to occur between 21 and 45 days apart.

She shouldn't require more than six to eight pads per day when she does get her period. She should consult a gynecologist or her doctor if she is filling up more frequently than that. While she might experience some cramping, intense pain that prevents her from going to school or participating in other activities isn't typical, so it's especially important to take note of.

For women, menstruating is a normal and essential part of life, but there is still shame associated with it. Girls frequently receive the message that having a period is something to be embarrassed about from boys who wince at the word "tampon" to commercials that appear uncomfortable to display the product they are offering.

Girls with ADHD may be especially sensitive to possible shame because they frequently struggle to fit in socially. Discussing menstruation openly and easily with your daughter will encourage her to have a healthier, more self-assured perspective on her body.

PMS & ADHD'S EMOTIONAL MESS

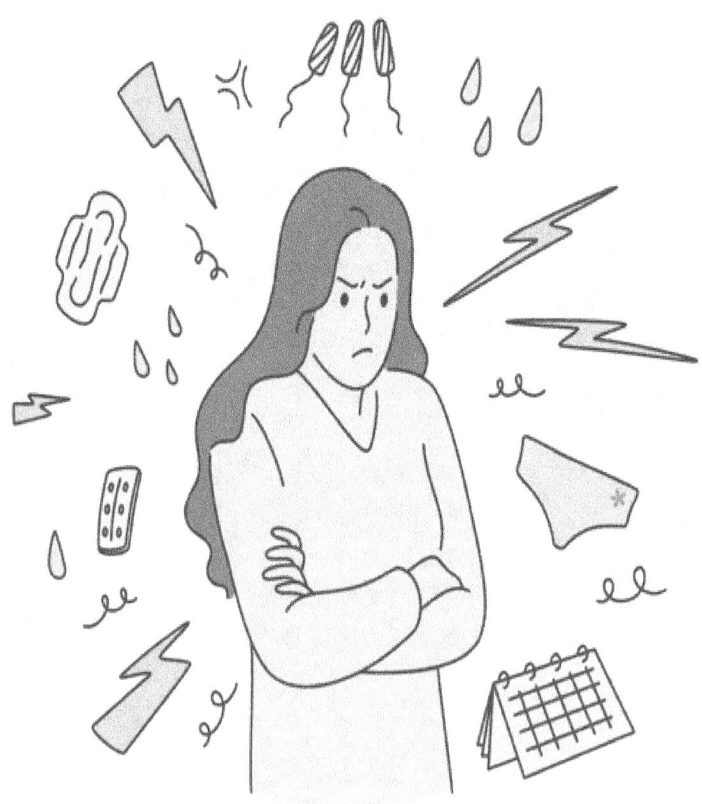

It's inevitable that teenage girls will experience emotional difficulties; it's just how the world is. There is a significant shift when ADHD is added on top of it. Even on their happiest days, girls with ADHD might experience difficulties. The premenstrual syndrome is then included.

According to Mandi Silverman, PsyD, the ups and downs of PMS can often be more severe for girls with ADHD. It can be extremely daunting for a girl who already struggles to control her emotions because it is so distracting. Getting your daughter ready is the greatest approach to help her deal with the uncomfortable feelings brought on by PMS. Have her make a chart showing the effects of her period over three cycles.

Your daughter will be able to make helpful changes once she starts to understand how her cycle affects her. This will allow her to be better prepared for issues like lack of focus or moodiness that frequently arise. According to Patricia Quinn, MD, author of "Understanding Women with AD/HD," fluctuations in estrogen levels during adolescence and again around menopause can have a significant impact on a woman's ADHD symptoms and daily functioning. Both a woman's premenstrual syndrome symptoms and her ADHD symptoms might get worse with similar changes in her menstrual cycle. Here are some things that could be useful:

- more physical activity and sleep
- Discuss with the teachers how to prepare in advance for a challenging day or days.
- Stop participating in social events.

- Look for stress-free, mindless distractions. ADHD medication and PMS while coloring and listening to music

PMS in people with ADHD generally seems to get worse at the end of the menstrual cycle. Girls may experience symptoms that are significantly stronger than usual in addition to seeing that their medication does not appear to be working as intended.

There is evidence, according to WebMD, that stimulants work more effectively when paired with estrogen. So, as those levels fall in the days preceding a period, girls may experience worsening symptoms. Several drugs are known to have negative effects, including but not limited to uncomfortable and painful periods. A doctor should be consulted on changing drug dosages during cycles.

Being a support system for your children
Making sure females are aware of their strong support systems would be beneficial at this period. Although a period is nothing to be embarrassed of, it is sometimes viewed as unpleasant or revolting. Although unpleasant, it is natural and shows how powerful and talented the female body is.

Young girls with ADHD who are going through this upheaval in their lives can feel less alone by having open and honest interactions with them. Sharing experiences, emotions, and questions with others makes it easier to know that they've been there too. Helping these young girls establish a routine and a sense of balance will ultimately be crucial. Her life will be made a lot simpler by this. They often have enough challenges to deal with, but with the correct support network and strategy in place, they won't have to fear their period as much.

How to Handle a Teen Who Is Extremely Emotional Because of PMS

Your mood can definitely be impacted by PMS. These tactics may be useful if you're having trouble with your teen's emotions during PMS.

Despite the fact that we frequently make light of premenstrual syndrome's moodiness. The fact is that PMS can impact your mood. Teenagers aren't free from this, which is unfortunate because parents sometimes find it challenging to deal with their mood swings.

These techniques may be useful if you're having trouble handling your teen's emotional problems brought on by PMS.

Encourage Your Teen To Go On Solo Trips

Teens with PMS may struggle greatly with irritability. Unfortunately, their heightened emotions can cause them to instigate confrontations with family members or act out of character around them. Because of this, the staff at Verywell Family advises adolescents to spend some time alone when they're feeling especially irate.

Your child can learn to control their emotions and calm down by spending time alone. Additionally, it might provide individuals with a secure setting in which to express repressed feelings like grief or self-consciousness. This provides them the chance to unwind and control the pain if they're experiencing weariness or cramping.

Time alone can also provide your child with a diversion, which can help them let go of their emotions. They have the option of reading a book, listening to music, playing a video game, or drawing. A nice distraction from impatience and other emotions is anything relaxing or enjoyable.

Encourage Them To Develop Healthy Habits

The Center For Women's Mental Health team at Massachusetts General Hospital claims that physical health issues, such as moodiness, can also affect PMS symptoms. In order to reduce some symptoms, it is probably a good idea to encourage them to adopt healthy habits.

Hormone balance and mood can be improved with proper eating. Hormone production is impacted by low levels of several vitamins as well as high quantities of salt and caffeine. Make certain that your youngster consumes balanced meals and limits their caffeine use.

Additionally, exercise helps improve their mood and lessen negative emotions like despair or rage. It doesn't have to be vigorous exercise; as part of your family's evening ritual, you can go for a stroll or do yoga. Moving even a little bit helps.

Avoid letting your emotions control you. At times during the month, it may seem like your teen is bothering you considerably more than usual (and maybe they are). But this too shall pass, just like every other stage you've experienced with your child.

 As a result, it's ideal if you roll with the punches and keep your emotions under control when these gloomy periods are happening.

Registered psychologist Louise Gleeson wrote in Today's Parent that youngsters begin to defy authority more frequently in their teenage years. In many situations, this is only a symptom of "growing pains," and

when their moodiness takes over, your teen
doesn't mean what they say.

Therefore, if you wish to prevail in this
situation, be composed and sensible. Quick
reactions are effective, especially when they
acknowledge and demonstrate empathy for
your child's feelings. Then, shift the
conversation and carry on. You can clear the
air if necessary once the storm has passed.
Every day dealing with a teen's emotions
can be challenging. But dealing with PMS's
intense emotional side effects is even more
difficult. It will be a lot simpler if you give
your teen some space and control her
emotions.

COULD PMS REALLY BE CURED?

Some remedies and medication for people with ADHD dealing with PMS.

*S*ome female patients with **ADHD** discover that their meds are less effective during their period. Make an appointment with your doctor to discuss the advantages and disadvantages of changing medication during her cycle if you see that your daughter's **PMS** and period symptoms are making it more difficult for her to manage her **ADHD.**

Women who have significant mood swings or **PMDD** may benefit from antidepressants. The most often used medications are SSRIs. To treat PMDD, however, additional antidepressants are often recommended. During the menstrual cycle or for 10 to 14 days before each period, certain antidepressants may be used.

Anti-anxiety drugs are among the other **PMS** remedies.

Natural Remedies for **ADHD** and **PMS**

Exercise

Exercise may improve your mood and help you stay awake. Regular exercise is necessary to get the advantages, not only when PMS symptoms arise. On most days of the week, aim for 30 minutes of moderate physical exercise. Exercise that is intense on fewer days may also be beneficial.

Stress Reduction

It's important to develop appropriate coping mechanisms for stress since **PMS** may lead to tension, anxiety, and irritability. Different approaches are effective for certain ladies. You may wish to give yoga, meditation, massages, journal writing, or just conversing with friends a try. Making sure you get adequate sleep also helps.

OTC Medicines

OTC painkillers help lessen some of the physical signs of **PMS**, including cramps, back discomfort, breast tenderness, and headaches. OTC medications that effectively treat these symptoms include Ibuprofen (Advil, Motrin, Midol Cramp)

Hormone Therapy

Hormone control is how birth control medications stop ovulation. This often results in lighter periods and may lessen **PMS** symptoms. Lupron, nafarelin, and other "GnRH" agonists, as well as synthetic steroids like danazol, are examples of further hormonal therapies. Before you locate one that relieves your symptoms, you may need to test a few other kinds.

The following vitamin and mineral supplements, according to studies, may lessen PMS symptoms:

Foods That Help:

B-Vitamin-Rich Diet

B vitamin-rich foods may aid in the treatment of PMS. More than 2,000 women were monitored by researchers for 10 years in one study. They discovered that women who consumed foods rich in thiamine and riboflavin, such as pork and Brazil nuts, were much less likely to have **PMS.** The same result wasn't achieved by using supplements.

Advanced Carbs

Complex carbohydrates rich in fiber include wholegrain, bread, and cereals. Fiber-rich foods may help you maintain stable blood sugar levels, which helps reduce mood swings and food cravings. Thiamine and riboflavin, two B vitamins that help prevent **PMS**, are also present in enriched whole-grain products.

Mint

Peppermint does more than simply make your breath fresh. In one trial, peppermint oil capsules were shown to be effective in treating IBS patients' stomach discomfort and other symptoms. Peppermint tea is OK to consume, but only the capsules have been shown to be effective. However, avoid it if you have heartburn since peppermint might aggravate it. Consult your physician before beginning any supplements.

Ginger

This plant root reduces bodily inflammation. Stomach and menstruation cramps could be relieved by doing this. Researchers discovered that taking a ginger supplement during the first three to four days of your cycle might lessen menstrual discomfort. Your stir-fries and sauces should include fresh or dried ginger. Alternatively, make ginger tea.

Tofu

Tofu is a wholesome food. According to research, calcium may reduce menstruation discomfort. That could be because the mineral promotes healthy muscle cell function. Tofu is loaded in calcium, just as milk, yogurt, and other dairy products are. There is enough firm tofu in half a cup to provide 25% of your daily requirements. Fortified orange juice and oatmeal are some more excellent options.

By consuming fewer of these items, you may be able to reduce **PMS** symptoms:

> By mySalt, which makes bloating more likely

- Caffeine, which may make you agitated
- Sugar, which may intensify desires
- Alcohol, which may be depressant

Fatty foods

Pass on the cheeseburger and fries if you are experiencing stomach ache. Fat takes longer for your body to digest, and it may induce cramps by causing your intestines to contract. Additionally, fatty diets may exacerbate irritable bowel syndrome (IBS). That is a digestive disorder that may affect 1 in 6 persons. Bloating, discomfort, constipation, and diarrhea may result from it.

Dairy Goods

Some individuals have stomach discomfort after consuming too much dairy. This is because milk contains a sugar called lactose, which is difficult for many people to digest. Within a few hours of eating, that may result in nausea, bloating, and stomach discomfort. It could be necessary to consume less milk, cheese, or other dairy products, while lactose-free options are also an option, as is taking an enzyme supplement.

Tea and Coffee

If you often have stomach discomfort, you may want to limit your intake of coffee, tea, and other caffeinated drinks. Because caffeine is a diuretic, you urinate more often. Additionally, caffeine may jangle your nerves and cause your muscles to tense up. Both of them have the potential to cause cramping.

Spicy peppers

Spicy food and an upset stomach often don't go along. Capsaicin is a substance found in chili peppers. In addition to making your mouth burn, it may also trigger stomach nerves and exacerbate cramping. As an example, studies reveal that eating a hot chili-based meal made persons with IBS sorer.

Fiber-Rich Cereal

A diet rich in fiber is often beneficial. Diabetes, heart disease, and weight gain may all be avoided with its aid. But a fast increase may cause or exacerbate stomach pains. Your body must adjust to digesting the tough material over time. Once you attain the recommended 25–35 grams per day, increase your intake of fiber by 3-5 grams each week.

Alcohol

Avoid drinking alcohol if you are experiencing menstruation cramps. Alcohol may prolong the pain, which explains why.

Diuretics cause you to urinate more often. Dehydration may result from this, which may worsen cramping. Additionally, drinking too much alcohol might drop your blood sugar, which could make you angrier than normal.

Sodium-Rich Foods

Americans consume too much salt,nine out of ten do. That may upset the balance of electrolytes, minerals that support proper muscular function. Your body may be more prone to cramping if you eat too much. You can get bloated as a result. Our diets mostly consist of things we buy at the supermarket or eat at restaurants. Check the salt content of food labels at the grocery store, and cook more regularly at home.

Effects of PMS on Other Conditions

PMS may make several chronic diseases' symptoms worse, including

1. Allergies and bronchitis
2. Anxiety and depression
3. Disorders or seizures
4. Migraines
5. If your illness worsens just before your period, be sure to tell your doctor.

PMS or Another Issue?

The symptoms of PMS may resemble those of other diseases or overlap with them, such as:

Anxiety or depression with menopause
syndrome of protracted weariness
thyroid condition
inflammatory bowel disease
The main distinction is that **PMS** symptoms change from month to month in a predictable way.

Tracking your symptoms to identify PMS

Keep note of your symptoms using a monitoring form like this one to determine if you have PMS. You could have PMS if you:

Symptoms start five days before to your menstruation.
Within four days after the onset of your cycle, symptoms disappear.
For at least three menstrual cycles, symptoms recur.

When to Visit a Physician
If you have any suicidal thoughts, call 911 or seek immediate medical attention. Additionally, if your symptoms are interfering with your everyday activities such as work, relationships, or other daily tasks, you should see a doctor immediately. This can be a symptom of PMDD, a more severe type of **PMS**.

Disorder of Premenstrual Dysphoria
The symptoms of the premenstrual dysphoric disorder (PMDD), which has the same pattern as **PMS**, are more

bothersome. Women who have **PMDD** may face difficulties that interfere with everyday living, such as panic attacks, weeping fits, thoughts of suicide, sleeplessness, or other issues. Fortunately, many of the methods used to treat **PMS** may also be used to treat **PMDD.**

A personal or familial history of depression, mental disorders, or trauma is one of the risk factors for PMDD.

CONCLUSION

A time of transition between childhood and maturity is adolescence. Children go through a lot of changes at this time of transition, both physically and mentally. One indication that a female has completed puberty is the onset of menstruation. A consistent flow of blood into the vagina from the uterine wall is known as menstruation. This shows that the female reproductive system has functioned. The interplay of hormones secreted by the hypothalamus, anterior pituitary, and ovaries affects menstruation. Women's cycles come in a variety of cycle variants.

Women have a variety of symptoms and menstruation throughout their periods. Physical discomfort or pains may manifest as both psychological and physical symptoms. beginning with symptoms of a tummy ache, breast pain, lightheadedness, nausea, sleeplessness, and irritability. Premenstrual syndrome (PMS) is the term used to describe this ailment, which may range from moderate to severe and call for medical attention.

They feel precisely gloomy, angry, or depressed as a result of these premenstrual symptoms. The women even have a sense of being in control, which has an impact on their interactions with husbands, coworkers, kids, and friends. Premenstrual dysphoric disorder is what this is (PMDD). Serious mental and physical issues linked to the menstrual cycle are part of the PMDD syndrome. After the midpoint of the menstrual cycle, the condition starts, and it stops when menstruation starts. Both PMDD and PMS have the same symptoms, such as sadness, anxiety, tension, and irritability, albeit the severity of each condition varies.

Student accomplishments and activities are significantly impacted by PMS.

 According to a study done at the Darul Arqam Islamic Boarding School, young ladies with significant amounts of body fat are a source of estrogen production, which makes PMS more prevalent in these women. Adolescent females often have the greatest symptoms of PMS, including trouble focusing and hip discomfort, which is the most common physical symptom. Young women who experience PMS have estrogen levels of 148.32, not 98.00 pg/ml as is often believed. A hormonal imbalance between estrogen and progesterone, where estrogen levels rise and serotonin synthesis declines cause PMS. This hormonal imbalance impacts mood and behavior. Prolactin, which may aggravate breast discomfort, and aldosterone, which contributes to salt retention, and air retention, which aggravates breast stress, can both be increased by excess estrogen.

Why Your PMS Cravings Are Perfectly Normal

The findings revealed that this impact of eating more was nevertheless felt by women who were not officially diagnosed with PMS. If you're a woman, you've probably had PMS cravings. Most women would confirm that it is true, cravings for chocolate or other foods may occur during their cycle depending on what our wacky hormones are telling us we need.

Sarah Twogood, an assistant professor of obstetrics and gynecology, examined the reasons why science demonstrates that these cravings are acceptable in an essay that was initially published on The Conversation. Evidently, along with mood swings and irritability, cravings are one of the most often reported signs of PMS (or premenstrual syndrome). It seems that women generally eat more during the part of their cycle before their menstruation.

Typically, we gravitate toward carbohydrates, lipids, and sweets (sounds about right). The findings indicated that women without a formal PMS diagnosis still experienced the effect of eating more, however, their diets appeared to be slightly different.

There are a few potential explanations for this, according to her research. Because carbohydrates can influence the quantity of serotonin released in the brain, it's possible that we seek out certain foods to improve our emotions. Researchers have also proposed that the desire to eat those delicious meals is motivated by hormones or by a desire to improve our mood appears to be true.

Whether or not they had received a PMS diagnosis, the women in this stage of their menstrual cycle appeared to be covered by the data she discovered. In order to help control these cravings and other premenstrual symptoms, Twogood's final piece of advice to women was to become familiar with their individual cycles and bodies. She also suggested taking steps to deal with PMS, noting that doing so can reduce the cravings that come along with it. Whatever the cause, it appears that these cravings are a completely normal and frequent aspect of the cycle. Perhaps even more natural than the cycle itself. So remember that you aren't being unreasonable the next time you have PMS and feel like you HAVE to have some chocolate. Simply put, you're listening to your cycle!

NOTES

NOTES